Important Legal Disclaimer:

Readers should be aware that the information contained within this book demonstrates the personal opinions of the author.

The information provided is not intended to be a substitute for medical advice. The author recommends that readers seek a medical consultation before embarking on any new exercise or nutritional program to ascertain that it is suited to individual needs.

It is advisable to seek the approval of your doctor prior to introducing any dietary changes that incorporate unfamiliar foods. The author has meticulously endeavoured to ensure the information provided in the book is accurate and in no way misleading.

The author cannot be held accountable for any damages or loss that ensue by the reader following the programs and advice outlined within the book, nor be held responsible for any damages or loss which ensue as a consequence of the actions recommended in the book.

The author provides this legal disclaimer to stress that all responsibility for the use of information within the contents of this book is assumed by the reader.

Table of Content

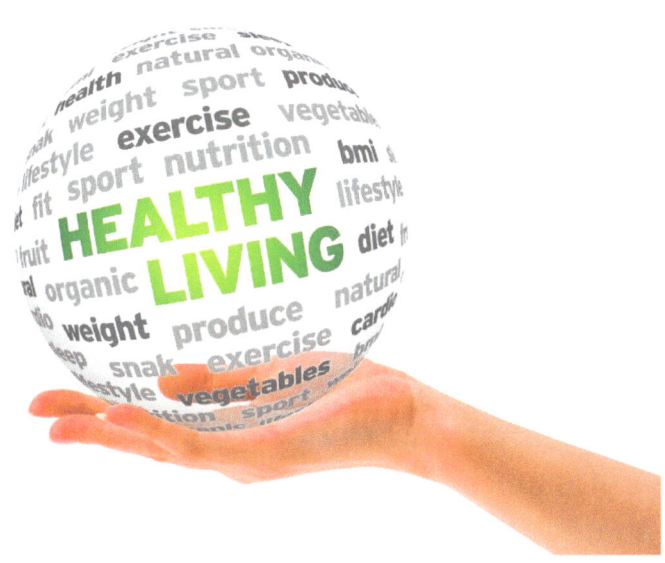

Introduction: What Are The Benefits Of Getting Slimmer With A Healthier And Safe Diet?

Slimming down is a process. It always has been and probably always will be. There are many things to consider; your health right now, your goals, your fitness levels and ultimately what you eat.

What we eat pretty much determines a large chunk of what fat goes where. A brief lesson in Biology is necessary to understand what happens when you eat and how your love handles and spare tires came to being.

A Brief Summary of Digestion

When you eat food, it is digested and the various nutrients are sent via the bloodstream to wherever they are needed.

Carbohydrates are energy-giving foods. For this reason, they have large amounts of sugar which is what provides the body with its energy.
If you have too much, you may end up having too much sugar in your bloodstream which may result in a sugar rush.

Your pancreas releases a hormone to neutralize this sugar and turn it into fat which is stored (in your thighs, arms, tummy etc) for later use. If you don't actually utilize this fat, it remains where it is and builds up over time.

When the body goes through starvation, the fats are broken down first. When there is no more fat to break down, the body then attacks the protein in your body which is your muscles for extra energy to keep itself running.

If you do introduce carbohydrates into your system again, your body will immediately store it away for emergency situations where it may have to starve again.

This is the reason starvation is not a good option for you. You may lose weight, but gaining it back is very easy and you may end up bigger than before.

Having a balanced meal and a healthy diet plan to compliment your exercise regimen is probably the safest way to lose weight.

This may include a few supplements, but there is a point to note here; your pills are ONLY supplements to the diet you are on and not the only important factor to it.

The purpose of diet pills is merely to provide your body with the nutrients and vitamins you are not otherwise getting.

Benefits of a health and safe diet for weight loss

So, if you are looking to shed some weight, what are the benefits of getting slimmer with a healthier, safe diet? Here are a few:

1. Effectiveness – There is a weird seesaw effect

that takes place when you starve yourself or eat a ridiculously tiny amount of food.

The moment you go off your diet or lose enough weight to make you confident enough to try carbs again, the fat will pile right on again.

Learning what to eat, how to eat it and when to eat it are important for you to make some helpful and permanent lifestyle changes. The weight will fall off and stay off as long as you eat right.

2. Overall Health – The fact is, you need food to survive. That is why it is a basic need. Your food serves various functions in the body.

Aside from giving you energy, you build muscle, you get warm, you feel better and you function at optimum levels all from the food you eat. While a lot of carbs will make you sluggish after a time, a little will give you just the right boost you need.

If you want more energy for longer, make sure you combine this with protein. Make sure you get your essential vitamins in too.

3. Safety – The safety aspect cannot be stressed enough when it comes to your diet. Not only will you be able to fully function on a healthy diet, but you can also avoid other diseases like hypoglycemia (type 2 Diabetes) and low blood pressure.

There is also the added risk of contracting rickets and goiter and scurvy on top of malnutrition.

Make sure you do proper research before you begin any diet; some may end up giving you health complications anyway.

4. Increased Energy – With the right kind of diet, you don't have to rely on coffee for that morning pick-me-up. You won't even need to hover around your kitchen so much anymore either.

The perfect diet will make you feel fuller and more energetic together with the workouts that you do. Coffee isn't so very bad for you, but that depends entirely on how much you are taking.

A bit of caffeine stimulates brain activity which is good.
If you find yourself living on eight cups of coffee daily just to keep your energy levels up, it may be time to cut back.

Fruit and smoothies are a great replacement and (after you get over the withdrawal symptoms) you will be much more grateful for it.

5. Recommended – Your diet, after consultation, will probably be the safest one for you. Consultation here will mean talking to a healthcare professional like your doctor, your nutritionist or your personal trainer.

No matter what it is you are planning to do, especially if you are trying to lose weight, they can provide you with the perfect diet plan.

Where some diets are focused mainly on protein intake and building of muscle, some people may be allergic to protein.

Mentioning this to the healthcare professional will help you come up with the best plan despite your condition.

6. Save Money – Some diet plans really don't work. Some you will have to spend a fortune on and they do not advocate for the safest and/or healthiest methods of weight loss.

After you have followed your diet for a while, you may notice a plateau or, after your diet, you may realize that your weight is coming back on again.

Save your money on plans that don't work, consult a professional and do proper research before you begin your plan.

7. Happiness – This may seem strange, but weight loss should actually be fun. It will be difficult going when you being but once you have a rhythm going, you should be able to actually look forward to your workouts.

The end result of weight loss will also make you happy if that was your goal in the first place.

You should not feel completely guilty when you have your first slice of cake in three months or when you have a small scoop of ice cream at the occasional birthday party. It is there for you to enjoy.

There are no "quick fixes" to health.
If you have spent ten, twenty years of your life in a state of carefree unhealthiness, it will obviously take time to undo the damage.

The trick is to go slow and to take things one day at a time. In the end, if you want to lose that weight and keep it off, a healthy diet is the way to go.

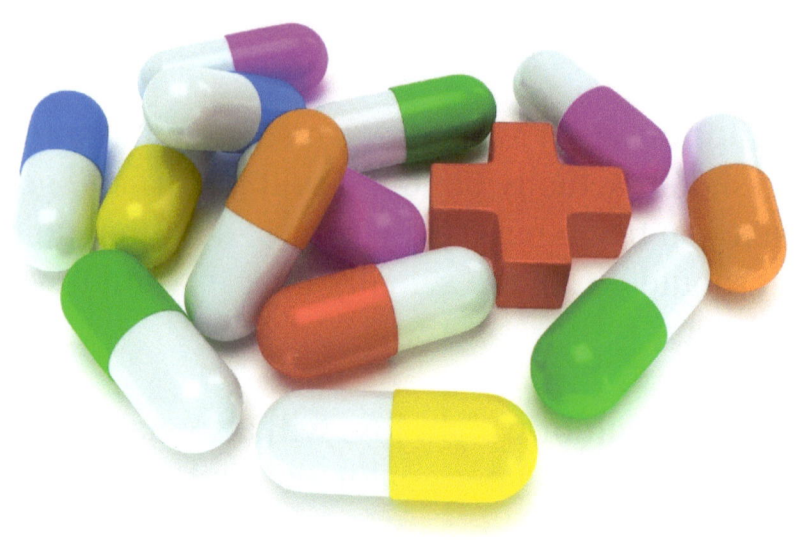

Diet Pills That Work

For the last so many years, there has been a bit of a health craze. Some people are looking for ways to get that pin-up body being advertised everywhere.

Others are looking to reverse the effects of lifestyle diseases they may have picked up along the way. Others still are simply out to be healthy and they feel they could stand to shed some weight.

Whatever the reason, many people have jumped onto the band wagon with a lot of pomp and vigor.

A bit about your diet pills

The mistake some people make is expecting that a particular plan will work like magic and one day they will just wake up tiny and toned and not have to worry about weight again.

There is really no such thing. Losing weight, getting fit and being healthy have no instant success secrets. Undoing all the years of unhealthy living you've had will not take two minutes of hard exercise.

And then in comes the diet pill – the most controversial part of the whole health world.

Diet pills should essentially only supplement a diet. The same way you need a basket to carry things on your bike but you don't really need to have one for you to ride.

Some diet pills provide us with extra supplements, vitamins and/or minerals that you would otherwise not be taking in due to your diet change or the amount of fat you will be losing as you exercise.

It is very important to do your research concerning diet pills. Some of them have really bad side effects that shouldn't, and in the long run cannot, be ignored.

The best way to make sure you are taking the right pills the right way is to consult a healthcare expert; your doctor, your nutritionist or even your personal trainer or fitness instructor could help you out here.

Popular diet pills and their effects

That being said, there is no doubt that there are some diet pills that actually fit the bill and do a good job, even in spite of their side-effects. Here are some effective diet pills, a brief description of how they work and some side effects you may encounter.

1. Xenical – This is a diet pill that should be taken with caution. Xenical works to burn away the fat inside of your body and expel it using the digestive tract.

This means that you will be getting oily stools depending on how much fat is contained in your food. On top of this, you may also experience gas and frequent bowel movements.

While taking Xenical, it is advisable to steer clear of foods with high fat content. There are some medical conditions that may be affected with the use of Xenical like a family history of stroke or heart disease.

This is a prescription drug. Do not buy it over the internet since you cannot be sure of the contents and they may bring you more harm than good.

2. D4 Thermal Shock – Thermal means heat. This diet pill works to raise your temperature which has been known to increase your rate of metabolism. This in turn burns calories and you lose weight.

This particular pill is more effective with exercise. Just like Xenical, however, you need to watch what you eat because it also produces oily stools.

Aside from this, the side effects you may experience include tingling (which may occur about half an hour to forty minutes after ingestion) and paranoia after taking a heavy dose over a long period of time.

3. Phentermine – This particular drug acts as an appetite suppressant. This means that you eat less and feel less hungry even as you do so allowing you to reduce the amount of food you eat and therefore have less calories in your system.

This in turn lets you burn more than you gain when you exercise. This pill also has side effects mostly centering around your heart rate and blood pressure. It is known to raise blood pressure so it will be dangerous for you if you have heart problems or high blood pressure.

4. Alli – It is a slightly more effective option than Phentermine which, instead of only suppressing your hunger, binds itself to your fat cells causing them to be more easily expelled from the body. Just like Xenical and D4, however, this pill also causes very oily stools which can easily turn to diarrhoea. It should be taken mostly with low-fat healthy meals to avoid this unpleasant side effect.

Some other side effects may include gas and cramping pains. Please consult your physician before you take it.

5. Hoodia – This particular drug has been in question for a long time, but it works in pretty much the same way as Phentermine.

It suppresses the appetite and reduces cravings meaning you won't be giving up at the end of the day of dieting and stocking up on carbs again.

It is an extract of a wild plant growing in South Africa that has been known to have these appetite suppression qualities. It also has no side effects so it is very safe to experiment with.

Summary and Conclusion

These are just five of possibly hundreds of diet pills out there that more or less work the same way as these ones. They suppress your appetite or make your body fat more soluble.

Some may end up becoming addictive and others are only supplements that you can either take or not take. Others still are taken to accelerate the effects of another supplement you are taking.

Whatever the case, there is no denying that diet pills can work for you.

The warnings on the boxes should not be ignored. Some could cause you some serious health problems.

It should be noted that weight loss while pregnant is very dangerous and even if you do need to lose weight, do so only under the doctor's instructions to ensure both your safety and that of your unborn child.

Also, make sure you do your research on a particular pill and beware of buying prescription pills online. It would be far much safer to buy your pills from your local pharmacy.

Although you will be spending a little more money, let's be honest; it's better to be safe now with a verified and certified bottle of pills than very sorry later with a bottle of pills whose contents have not and cannot be verified and/or approved by a medical professional.

There is no "miracle pill" per se that will let you carry on your current unhealthy lifestyle (no diet or exercise) that will still let you lose weight. You have to be willing to work for it.

If you see a drug that sounds way too good to be true, it probably is and therefore isn't worth your time. ALWAYS make sure you are using your diet pill as a compliment to a diet and not as the main/only component of your dieting.

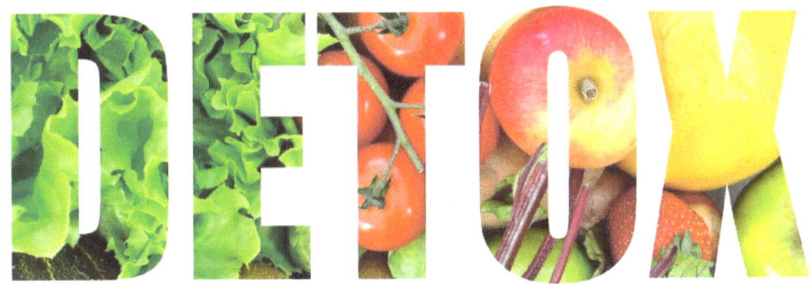

Diet Meal Plans (Paleo Cleanse And Detox)

In today's highly enlightened world, more and more individuals are taking the necessary time and resources to ensure that they consume the right kinds of food.

As would be expected there are happen to be diverse diets that have been touted as been in a position to present plenty health, fitness and wellbeing benefits.

Which range from effectual weight loss and

maintenance, prevention of diseases as well as revitalizing the body and its critical organs.

The following happens to be an in-depth review of 3 diet meal plans (paleo, gluten-free, cleanse and detox) that can go a long way in permitting you to achieve your health and fitness objectives.

The paleo diet

To begin with, the paleo, or if you like, caveman diet is undoubtedly one of the most popular meal plan in existence. It is founded on the purported eating habits of our hunting and gathering ancestors who lived in the Paleolithic period.

This diet comprises of foods that can be hunted or fished (meat and seafood) as well as those that can be gathered such as eggs, fresh fruits, vegetables spices and herbs.

And excludes cereal grains, potatoes, refined/processed foods and salt. In essence the paleo diet happens to be a low carbohydrates, high protein meal plan that is characterized by making ideal variations in carbs and meat consumption.

Most of its supporters assert that such a balance of

food consumption offers diverse long-term health benefits.

That can play a crucial role in assisting sustainable weight loss and decreasing the risks of contracting serious diseases like diabetes, heart disease and even cancer.

Which is brought about by sticking to a diet that consists of less processed foods, and eating plenty of fresh vegetables as well as fruits. The paleo diet is also highly noted for its unmatched simplicity, and does not in any way require calories counting.

An ideal paleo meal plan demands a lot of home cooking, but you can circumvent this by integrating a weekly cook-up day where you can conduct your shopping and batch cooking for an entire week.

It is also important to make a suitable paleo meal template you can use as a guiding beacon to integrate and variate recipes to eliminate monotony. You should also stick to ingredients that are easily accessible.

The gluten-free diet

For those who may be perhaps not in the know, a gluten-free meal plan excludes the consumption of the protein gluten that is found in grains such as wheat, barley and rye.

This kind of diet is primarily geared for individuals that have celiac disease (gluten intolerance), which triggers small intestine inflammation. It hence enables such people to effectually manage the signs and symptoms of this ailment as well as curbing the risk of complications.

Additionally, this diet can be ideal not only for individuals that suffer from gluten intolerance, but also those that have difficulties in regulating their blood sugar levels, fat loss and increasing their energy levels.

Naturally, adhering to a gluten-free diet is extremely challenging. But with some fortitude and ingenuity, you will be able to discover that there are many foods that you already consume which are gluten-free.

As well as identifying viable alternatives for the gluten-rich foods you enjoy eating. Some of the foods that are naturally gluten-free include unprocessed beans, seeds (pumpkin and sunflower), nuts, fresh vegetables and fruits, fish and poultry (unmarinated, unbreaded, uncoated and unbuttered).

Grains and starches such as sorghum, millet, rice, corn, cornmeal, brown lentils and even seaweed. Together with foods with high fiber content that effectively curbs gluten-rich foods cravings.

An appropriate gluten-free meal plan should consist of incorporating the above mentioned foods into breakfast, mid-morning snack (ideally a whole fruit), lunch, mid-afternoon snack and a large dinner.

The cleanse and detox diet plan

Cleansing as well as detoxifying meal plans have over the recent years become extremely popular, most especially with the endorsements from many celebrities.
These kinds of diets are deemed to present a plethora of health and fitness benefits, top among them been the comprehensive elimination of toxins from the body.

Some of them are also feted as been in a position to regulate the wellbeing and functionality of critical body organs such as the liver and large intestine. As well as regulating blood sugar levels, blood pressure, insulin levels and even blood cholesterol levels.

One popular cleansing and detox diet happens to be the liver cleanse, which avoids foods and beverages that have high concentrations of fructose, hydrogenated oils, food additives and preservatives.

That are then replaced with organic and free-range foods such as broccoli, kale, Brussels sprouts, cauliflower and even cabbage.

All of which are widely acclaimed for possessing some sulphur compounds which go under the name glucosinolates that effectually bind on toxins in the liver and eliminate them.

The liver cleanse also disapproves of salt and flavor foods (garlic, rosemary) consumption, both of which have been established to trigger fluid retention in the body.

On the other hand, the master cleanse happens to be another extremely popular cleansing and detox meal plan that is particularly thought to be excellent in facilitating rapid weight loss.

Following this diet essentially means swapping solid meals with a concoction that consists of lemon water, maple syrup and cayenne pepper.

Together with consuming a herbal detox tea on a daily basis for at least ten days.

Finally, the juice cleanse is also an especially excellent cleansing meal plan. It simply entails replacing solid meals with juiced fresh vegetables and fruits.
Which also enables you to get plenty of crucial vitamins and minerals without having to consume a lot of whole fruits and vegetables.

Typically, you can opt for either a three day or seven day juice cleanse (or fast as it is sometimes called). And all you will need to invest in is appropriate fresh fruits as well as vegetables and an excellent juicer.

All in all, following these diet meal plans (paleo, gluten-free, cleanse and detox) can enable you to enhance your health, fitness and vitality in a very hassle-free manner.

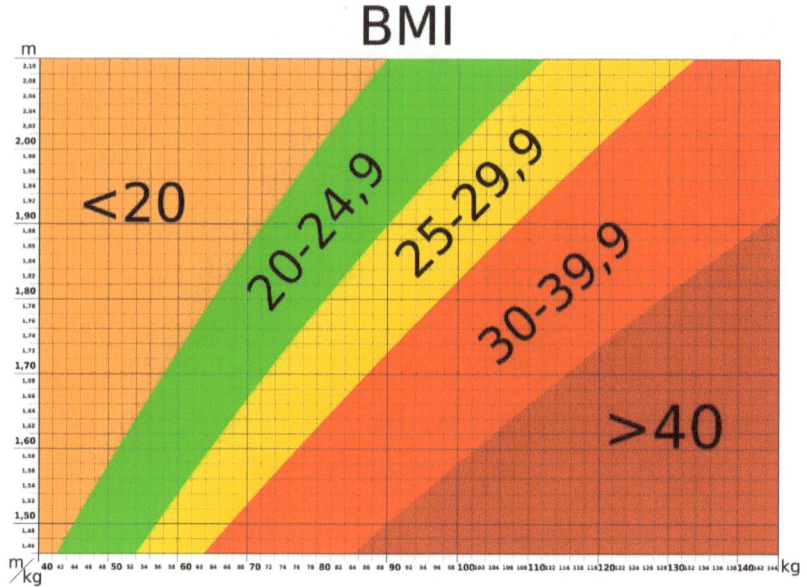

Diet For High Blood Pressure Patients

High blood pressure which is also known as hypertension can be through the use of a good diet plan. The condition can be controlled using medication; however, a change in diet will make managing this condition even easier.

With a good diet, one may not even need to take as much medications and the benefits of the diet may include having the medication being more effective.

Reduce intake of sodium

A high blood pressure diet requires minimum sodium rich foods. Sodium can be reduced by minimizing intake of processed foods, being keener on the ingredients used to make the foods you purchased and keeping a record on how much sodium you are taking.

Sufficient potassium in the body helps to keep the levels of sodium low as sodium has been known to raise blood pressure. Magnesium also produces the same benefits. For this reason, foods with both minerals will be very effective in reducing the blood pressure.

Taking foods rich in potassium is more advantageous than taking potassium supplements. However, whichever source one chooses, should be with the help of their doctor.

Spices and herbs such as ginger, rosemary and cinnamon can in addition be integrated into the recipes especially with the vegetables and soups. The use of sodium in food can be replaced with the use of spices such as garlic.

What to include in your diet for high blood pressure:

*Grains and nuts

*Grains such as pasta, cereals, bread and rice

Whole grains contain fiber and are more nutritious than the processed ones. Grains do not contain too much fat which makes them ideal for those wanting to keep their weight level. The best grains are brown rice, whole grain bread and whole wheat pasta.

Although nuts will also be rich in the minerals necessary to lower blood pressure, they have high calorie content too.

Other nutritious benefits of nuts include omega 3 fatty acids and amino acids from certain types of nuts. Unsalted sunflower seeds are a good source of magnesium making it a healthy snack.

Vegetables and fruits

Vegetables are rich in vitamins, minerals and fibers. Some of these include sweet potatoes, carrots and broccoli. They contain magnesium and potassium which are necessary when lowering the level of blood pressure.

Combine vegetables into your recipes to ensure that you have enough daily supply.

Highly consider green leafy vegetables such as spinach as they rich in folate besides magnesium and potassium. They also have a lot of fibers and few calories which are important in keeping blood pressure at a regulated level.

Most of the fruits will not have a high content of fat and just like the vegetables; they are rich in fiber and minerals.

One can take fruits as a healthy snack or combine them with a meal. The peelings from some of these fruits are also quite nutritious for instance those from apples and pears.

When taking packed vegetables, check whether they have salt additives or sodium and avoid those with these additives. For fruits that have been canned, select those without additional sugar.

Additionally, ensure that you let your doctor know of the fruits you intend to include in your meals as some of the fruits will react with the high blood pressure medications.

Sweets and chocolate

Do not take too many sweets especially those

containing too much sugar and fat. Dark chocolate with cocoa power will also help reduce the level of blood pressure On the other hand, do not take it in excess as it contains a lot of calories.

Take the right beverages

Remember to drink plenty of water. Other healthy drinks include low fat yogurt which is very nutritious as it contains proteins, vitamin D and calcium.

Although the studies on the effects on caffeine on blood pressure are not quite as in-depth, do not take caffeine in excess.

One can monitor their changes in blood pressure as they consume caffeinated drinks to determine it has any effect on them and how large this effect is.

Management of weight is really crucial when it comes to lowering blood pressure. This will be done effectively by the adoption of a healthy diet. This includes a food plan with low calorie levels.

Alcohol contains calories therefore; a high intake will result to weight gain. It will in addition raise the blood pressure levels and will in addition have negative effects on the cardiovascular and neurological system.

Meat and dairy products

Another source of calcium is lean meat and in addition contains iron and vitamins B. Take lean meat in moderation taking care to minimize having to fry them in fat.

When you choose to consume dairy products, select those whose fat content is low. Consume poultry, fish and whole grains at a moderate level.

Varieties of beans such as kidney, black, navy, white and lima beans will have the magnesium and potassium needed to reduce blood pressure levels. What's more, it has soluble fiber to improve the overall health.

Fats

Choose foods with the right kind of fats. Although fat is necessary to strengthen the immune system help the body to utilize the necessary vitamins, chose those with saturated fats instead of those with Trans fats.

Saturated fats will be contained in such foods as

palm oil, butter and red meat which will increase the level of cholesterol in the body.

Poly unsaturated fats found in such oils as sunflower, rapeseed and olive oil will reduce cholesterol levels. Despite this, one should still not take them in excess are they are likely to cause weight gain.

How to maintain a good high blood pressure diet

Keep a record of what you eat. This will help you know where you have been going wrong and the changes you need to make.

Avoid impulse buying of foods without nutritional value by planning your food shopping before purchase. Also ensure to read the label on foods before purchasing them to ensure that they have the valuable content you need for your high blood pressure diet.

Adopt the new diet gradually. This will make it easiest for you to adjust and follow through with the adjustments.

Get social supports from those also trying to lower their blood pressure using diet. This will keep you motivated in following through with your change in meals.

Always consult your medical practitioner before making any dietary changes. Also, ensure that you always take your hypertension medication unless advised otherwise by your doctor.

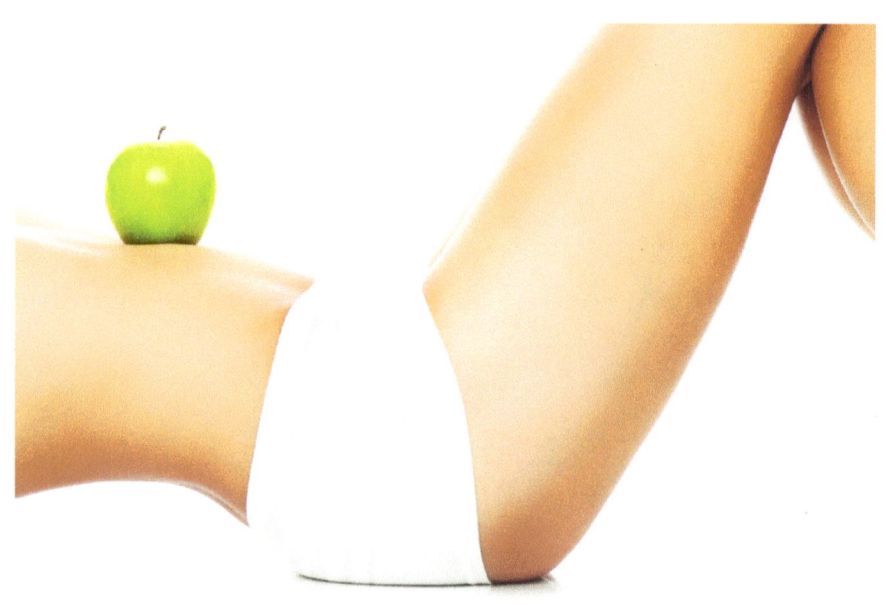

Diets To Lose Weight Fast

Perhaps the most irritating part about weight loss is all the methods that can work. Quite literally, if you ask ten different people how to lose weight you may get fifteen different answers.

It's all a bit crazy and can be really frustrating to some which is why some people like to just forget about it altogether.

The diet fads are another thing. One moment this food is banned and tagged as terrible for your health and the next, it's the best thing you could eat. There is no end to it at all.

Not to mention that some food requirements can just be downright nasty (for you at least; some people like raw carrot with steamed cauliflower).

Basically it all just comes down to eating a lot less and moving a lot more. Regardless of what diet you are following (as long as you aren't starving yourself) you should be having three square meals a day (with or without snacks depending on your diet) and a strict exercise regimen to keep.

Dieting can only take you so far but hand in hand with exercise, you can get yourself back in shape in almost no time.

Some quick weight loss diets

If you are looking to lose weight quickly, there is really no "instant solution." You have to do it the hard way and work for it and probably give up a few things you love (that pizza slathered in cheese and deep fried meat for example).

Here are a few diets that, according to their reviews, actually work for some people and help them lose weight fast:

1. Dr. Oz's 2 week Rapid Weight Loss Diet – This plan has seen viewers lose quite a bit of weight in only two weeks. It involves a bit of a radical lifestyle change especially where eating is concerned.

The basics are cutting out foods that make you fat (like dairy and wheat) and eat unlimited quantities of low glycemic foods which will promote faster fat burning.

Then you will also need to take probiotics nutrients which more or less speed up your weight loss.

2. The 7 day 1200 calorie meal plan – This plan works to help you eat less in a week. Less calories means less fat being stored in your body and therefore more weight loss.

Eating smaller meals is the main trend and while you do get a smaller serving that you usually would, you can still enjoy foods like Cheerios and waffles albeit in controlled amounts.

Over 90 days, you should have lost quite a bit of weight and gotten into the habit of eating lighter caloric meals which more or less help you reach your daily weight loss goals.

3. 3 step weight loss plan – This one is not so much a diet as a plan which features three crucial steps to weight loss; eliminating sugars and starches (carbohydrates), eating protein, vegetables and fat (yes, you read right – fat) and exercising 3-4 times a week.

Of course eating fat doesn't mean chugging down a cup of oil every day (which is pretty nasty). You can get your fats in healthy ways from coconut oil or olive oil used in dressing or cooking and even from butter.

By removing carbs from the diet, you are allowing your body to use up its stored resources and build muscle instead of fat.

4. The Dukan Diet – This one is also based on low carb intake and high protein intake. It is important to note that for the first week, you do not have any carbohydrates, some vegetables and all fats completely.

For the next part, the diet reintroduces these components into your diet in small amounts. While this diet promotes quick weight loss, you may experience bad breath, dizziness, nausea and even insomnia from cutting out carbohydrates in the first week.

Since it does not involve counting calories, this is a bonus since you just eat what is acceptable.

5. The Atkins Diet – This diet seems to be the one that started it all. When Atkins was diagnosed by his doctor with obesity, he was given a weight loss plan which then went on to take the world by storm.

While it focuses on also cutting out a lot of carbohydrates in the first phase, it doesn't cut them out completely. Also in contrast, it does allow for vegetables and fat.
After this, carbohydrates and fruit are introduced back in your diet allowing you to make use of its energy instead of storing it in your body as fat.

This diet also does not include calorie counting (which is rather tedious) but instead allows for quick weight loss as long as you follow the rules.

6. The Cambridge Diet – This diet promotes mea-replacement products for weight loss. Depending on your diet goals and for a more long term effect, you can have a plan ranging from 415 to 1500 calorie intake in one day.

Together with your low calorie meals, you are allowed to take some bars, shakes and porridges that compliment your diet and give you added nutrition.

The weight loss in this case is usually astonishingly rapid but side effects could include tiredness, dizziness, insomnia and bad breath among others.

Also, swapping meals for a snack bar or shake can make office lunch hour pretty boring and you can start feeling left out. This is one plan that you will have to try very hard to stick to.

7. Slim Fast Diet – This meal plan switches out your normal meals with lower calorie ones to help you lose weight fast. It is most effective for those who have a BMI of 25 and above.

This diet advocated for use of Slim Fast products and three snacks a day (including chocolate – yay!) in addition to your low calorie meals. There are no forbidden foods and no calorie counters involved which makes it easy to follow.

Some of the requirements may be harder to come by like the large amounts of fruit a protein but if you get it right, you can follow it easily and lose weight.

One other important drawback is that it is easy to gain weight once you stop the diet and stop using the products. The diet itself doesn't teach you much about healthy living.

There are hundreds of diets to lose weight fast out there each with their own pros and cons. In the end, you need a plan that will work best for you and your doctor, nutritionist and/or personal trainer may be able to help you get the right one for you.

The two most important rules of diet plans are simple; too good to be true may not be as good as it sounds and when in doubt, always consult a healthcare specialist.

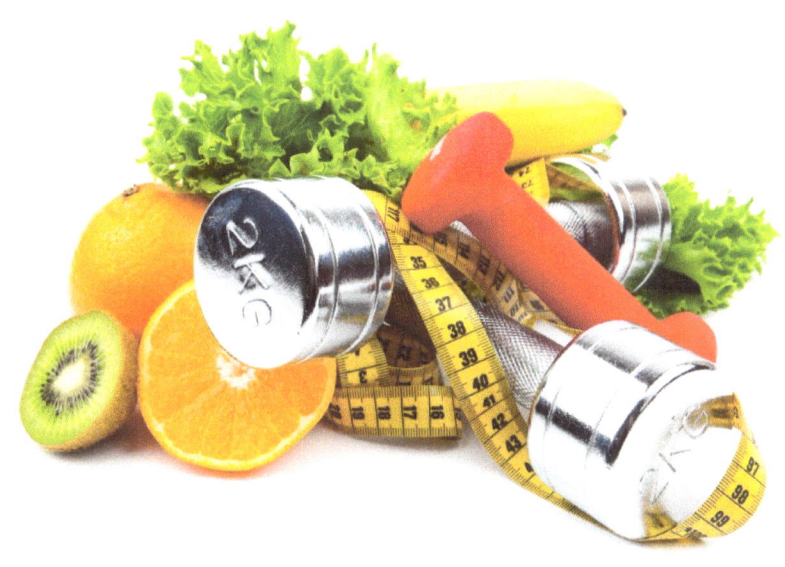

Top Diet And Exercise Plans Recommendations

As would be expected health and fitness spheres, all over the world, are awash with a multitude of diet and exercise plans you can opt for.
Many of which sadly fail to deliver on the glittering promises their creators offer.

However, there are fortunately still other excellent dieting and workout programs that have been firmly established to facilitate for rapid fat loss, significant muscle gain as well as boosting general health and fitness levels.

Indeed, there happen to be even diet and exercise plans that have been known to greatly reverse the physical manifestations of the aging process.

Which can naturally go a long way in enabling you to appear up to a decade younger than you really are.

The right exercise program accelerates the fat burning process and muscle growth

Typically, an ideal exercise regimen should effortlessly integrate effectual fat burning that, of course, targets the most problematic regions of the body such as the tummy, thighs and even buttocks (women).

While also facilitating for building of lean muscles that can be indispensable in boosting your metabolism for optimal round the clock fat burning.

Effectual dieting goes hand in hand with working out to achieve better outcomes

Additionally, while undertaking such an exercise regimen, you should also closely watch your eating habits. It is essential to feed your body with the right kind of nutrients, most especially proteins that happen to be the building blocks of muscles.

What types of proteins are ideal for a comprehensive diet and exercise plan?

Ideally, you should consume foods rich in proteins in every single meal you take as they provide the body with the amino acids that are necessary for maximum muscle toning.

According to your gender and even preferences you can include appropriate amounts of skinless poultry, lean beef (tenderloin, roast or even sirloin) and seafood (fresh, canned or frozen) into every meal you have each day.

The top diet and exercise plans also supplement animal-based proteins with vegetable alternatives to offer the body a much broadened spectrum of this invaluable nutrient.

Eat plenty of fruits and vegetables

It is also important to include at least one serving of fresh or frozen fruits as well as vegetables in each meal you take.
Doing this will ensure that your body is adequately supplied with the ideal nutrients (vitamins and minerals) to replenish those depleted by your

workout regimen. While at the same time also boosting your general health, energy levels and wellbeing.

Fruits and vegetables, through their antioxidant properties, also play a critical role in the fighting of free radical formation in your muscle cells that characterizes plenty of high intensity exercises.

Eat more wholesome snacks

You should also make it a point to integrate snacks such as unsalted nuts and edible seeds at least two times each day.

Given, these types of food contain fat and loads of calories, but they also happen to be excellent sources of protein, essential fats, fiber and plenty of antioxidants.

The latter of which are also indispensable in combating the kind of inflammation that wrecks havoc on your skin, which usually leads to wrinkling and other manifestations of aging.

One thing to take note of when integrating nuts and seeds into your diet plan is to always settle for low-calorie alternatives such as almonds as opposed to high-calorie ones like brazil nuts.

The latter of which can make the whole weight loss initiative rather counterproductive.

Avoid dairy and soy products and opt for whole grain foods

It is also highly recommended to steer clear from dairy and soy products in your dieting and exercising regimen. Which have been known to trigger food sensitivity that often leads to bloating as well as diminished energy levels.
As you progress in whatsoever diet and exercise plans you opt for, you can begin to integrate at least 100 calories per meal of whole grain products.

Such as multigrain bread, oatmeal, whole wheat pasta and even brown rice. All of which can come in handy in boosting your energy levels, providing your body with the nutrients it needs and keeping you satiated for longer in between meals.

Steer clear from processed foods and take an ideal multivitamin supplement

On the other hand, you should avoid consuming processed foods most of which can contribute to the kind of inflammation that fast-tracks the aging process.

Finally, you can supplement your regular meals with a daily dose of a potent multivitamin product to boost your overall health and vitality.

This should include at least 350 mg to 500 mg of calcium, which is especially excellent in building strong and healthy bones. As well as about 200 mg to 400 mg magnesium, which aids in effectual calcium absorption in the body.

Let us now take a closer look at the ideal workout regimen you can incorporate into your lifestyle.

Opt for cardio and strength training for effectual fat burning and muscle toning

When it comes to highly effective exercises, particularly for weight loss, cardiovascular workouts that are combined with moderate strength training are the most utilized in diet and exercise plans that produce results.

Cardios such as biking, swimming, jogging and even walking play a critical role in increasing your heart rate, which in extension leads to accelerated fat burning.

To this end, it is critical to integrate at least twenty minutes of cardio workouts schedules for five days every week.

While also undertaking restful strengthening and body conditioning exercises like moderate free weight training that will infinitely boost your body's metabolism.

Integrate interval training into your workout schedule

To further heighten the effectiveness of such an exercise program, you should also incorporate appropriate interval training.

Which basically should consist of mixing high as well as low intensity workouts at the rates recommended above. But also making sure you provide for adequate rest periods in between.

Conclusion

Following these diet and exercise plans suggestions can be the turning point you need to gain the health, fitness and wellness objectives you might have set up for yourself. And one might add, in a totally sustainable, convenient, time effective and stress-free manner.

Diet Supplements 101: All You Need To Know About This Products

For those who may perhaps not be in the know, diet supplements are products whose formulation comprises of various ingredients such as vitamins, minerals, herbs, amino acids and even enzymes that present health benefits.

Typically, these products are specifically designed to enable their users to have sufficient intake of the above mentioned nutrients that the body needs to carry out its functions.

This means that they are geared to supplement a diet and hence can contain one or more dietary ingredients or in some cases, even their constituents.

However, this doesn't mean that these products can replace foods that are critical in a healthy diet.

In essence diet supplements are, for the most part, taken orally and come in diverse forms like capsules, powder, tablets, liquid, soft gel or even gelcap formulation.

Diet supplements are not strictly regulated as medicines

In most countries, makers of these products are obligated by the law to make sure that they are safe for human consumption. And the information supplied on their labels is accurate and not in any way misleading.

Nevertheless, taking a case study of the US, the FDA, which is responsible for regulation of diet supplements, doesn't require manufacturers to provide data on their safety before they are available in the market.

Which is undoubtedly a sharp contrast from the strict regulations that are enforced on medicinal drugs.

Diet supplement manufacturers are permitted to make claims on their effectiveness before these products are subjected to scientific analysis Additionally, these firms are permitted to make health, structural/function and even nutrient content claims.

That elaborate on the link between these products and a food substance, disease or medical condition, health benefits and even concentration of a nutrient/s or dietary substance found in them.

Once diet supplements hit the market, the FDA usually analyzes their safety standards by conducting research as well as closely monitoring side effects reports from consumers and healthcare professionals.

In the event that such a product is found to be unsafe, the FDA can then take legal action on the manufacturer or even issue a warning on its usage and ban it.

Always take the time to review diet supplements before commencing to use them

To this end, it is highly recommended to get in-depth information like the effects and potential side effects on any dietary supplement you may wish to use.

You can consult your physician about diet supplements, and even if he/she may not be conversant with a particular product.

They may still be in an excellent position to easily access up to the minute medical data on its usage and associated health risks.

Consult your doctor if you are taking other medication

You should also seek medical clarification if you happen to be on any medication be it prescription or over the counter. Some of these products interact adversely with certain drugs.
You should also consult your primary healthcare provider should you be thinking of replacing your current medication with one or more dietary supplements.

Consult your physician before using diet supplements if you are about to have surgery/ pregnant, nursing a baby or intending to give these products to your child

The same applies if you are scheduled to undergo a surgical procedure. Some dict supplements have been found to enhance the risks of excessive bleeding as well as negatively influence the body's natural response to anaesthesia.

Should you be pregnant or nursing a baby or perhaps keen on giving your child any of these products, it is highly advisable to first get medical clearance from your doctor.

This is largely due to the fact that many of these products haven't been tested on pregnant, nursing mothers and even children.

Determine if diet supplements can complicate your medical condition

Should you have a certain medical condition it is also crucial to discover if the dietary supplement you want to take poses any risks to your ailment.

There are some diet supplements that have been established to give rise to even life threatening complications in individuals with certain medical conditions.

For example, diet supplements whose formulation contains iron are not safe for usage by persons with hemochromatosis. Which happens to be a hereditary disease that is characterized by excessive accumulation of iron in the body.

Taking such products can complicate matters as well as heightening the risks of contracting liver disease for individuals with this medical condition.

Not all natural diet supplements are safe for use

You should also be extremely wary of diet

supplements whose labels claim they are formulated from totally natural ingredients. Which doesn't always mean they are safe for consumption.

Some herbal varieties of these products are manufactured with many compounds, and not all of them might be known. On the other hand, some diet supplements may be formulated from the wrong plant species.

And at other times the exact concentration of the various natural ingredients may be lower or higher than the amounts stated on their labels.

In other circumstances these types of diet supplements can be contaminated by other botanical substances, metals and even pesticides. Or in some extreme scenarios, adulterated with unspecified illegal ingredients such as prescription medicine.

Review scientific based studies on diet supplements

To comprehensively access further information on these products, you can visit the websites of the national center for complementary and alternative medicine (NCCAM), the national institute of health (NIH) as well as other related federal agencies.

All of which offer free scientific publications and additional in-depth resources on many kinds of diet supplements that are currently available in the market.

Conclusion

All in all, after ascertaining the properties of a dietary supplement you wish to integrate into your diet, it is extremely important to follow the manufacturer's or even your physician's instructions to the letter.

Which can go a long way in enabling you to avoid any side effects or complications that can arise with using it.

Finally, should you experience any health problems after beginning to use diet supplements you should at once stop further intake and consult your doctor as soon as possible.

The above is an insight with this regard.

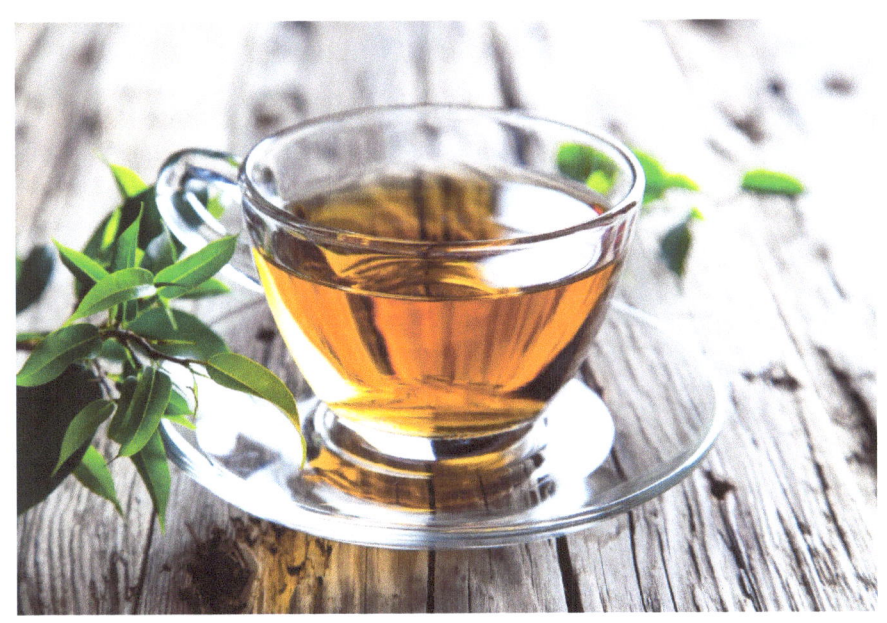

The Basics About Diet Tea

How to choose diet tea?

Diet tea comes in numerous varieties from green diet tea, Chinese diet tea, herbal diet tea and so much more. Ensure to select one that best matches your needs and does not pose a risk to your health.

These teas vary in form of taste and benefits. While some will be bitter and too strong others are flavored to make them sweeter. Some of the teas are also made with specific health purposes for instance; some of the diet teas are specifically for weight loss.

Consider the content if the tea. Diet teas containing aloe, rhubarb root, castor oil and senna will have laxative properties. This could have benefits such as promotion of weight loss or negative effects such as the reduction of potassium in the intestinal system.

Some of the best diet teas are those whose ingredients used in the product are natural. Check for those with too much additional sweeteners and avoid them.
Some of the natural ingredients used to sweeten the tea are spearmint, lemon, peppermint and cinnamon.

Benefits of diet tea

Those using it in effort to lose weight have recorded quicker progress when compared to those not using it. This tea does not contain as much calories as that which is present in most of the other teas.

Some of the diet tea used for weight loss will in addition contain guidelines on the kind of diet to take to effectively lose weight as well as the exercise plan that will be best combined with the tea for maximum benefits.

On the other hand, the use of laxatives for weight loss is not as effective as it will not have long term benefits.

The reduction of cholesterol levels in the body with diet tea intake then makes it possible to prevent cardio vascular illnesses too. It also does this by thinning blood and relaxing the blood vessels.

This herbal tea has also been used to cleanse the body getting rid of toxins. Senna contained in most of these teas boosts the contractions in the intestines causing more fluids to be produced by the colon.

Diet tea is also ideal for improving the metabolism and having one feel more energized and relaxed.

Some of the ingredients used in diet tea

This tea may contain only herbs some include licorice root which has anti bacterial properties and hibiscus. It in addition contains spices used mostly for flavoring the tea.

A number of of the teas also contain agar together with methylcellulose which are intended to make the user feel full thus reducing their appetite. This then helps to promote weight loss.

Leaves from the Chinese mallow are dried and crushed for use in the tea for its diuretic effects. It has in addition been in use for medical benefits for thousands of years.

Also used as a laxative Chinese mallow has the ability assist in treating kidney problems. It is in addition not recommended for those taking diabetes medication or those who are expectant.

This tea also contains vitamin c and polyphenols which have anti oxidant properties. This makes the tea able to reduce the chances of developing degenerative medical conditions.

Chrysanthemum is also one of the key ingredients in diet tea for its refreshing feel and health benefits. Some of these include improving the flow of blood, reducing the symptoms of colds and hypertension as well as improving eye and respiratory health.

Allergies such as those of ragweed should be considered before taking diet tea containing Chrysanthemum. It stimulates the brain and keeps the nerves relaxed.

Precautions when taking diet tea

Individuals suffering from diseases related to the gastro intestinal system should avoid taking the tea because of the senna contained in it.

Senna which is also known as Cassia Angustifolia should not be used by people with diarrhea or pain in their abdominal section as it may become worse upon drinking this tea.

Those taking medication should always consult their doctors before taking any diet tea. Mothers who are nursing or those who are expectant and advised to consult their medical practitioners before taking the tea as well.
Children are also not advised on taking the tea. This however depends on the kind of tea as they will have it indicated on the instructions.

Some of the manufacturers of tea may mislead customers by labeling their tea as diet tea or Chinese diet tea just for the purpose of making sales.

For this reason, when purchasing diet tea, ensure to go for a well known and quality brand. In addition, research more on what other customers who have used the product have to say about it before making a purchase.

Most importantly, let your doctor know before beginning to use the tea.

How to effectively use diet tea

The best time to take the tea in the morning is before having breakfast. Place the tea bag into the cup of hot water for more than two minutes. Some of the diet tea bags will need one to have them in water for three minutes and will need to be pressed and stirred too.

During lunchtime, take the tea before your meal without having to finish the entire cup. The tea can also be taken later in the evening right before going to bed.

One does not have to combine the tea with anything. Diet tea should especially not be taken with milk. Milk has been found to reduce the effectiveness of tea when it comes to breaking down fat.

Diet tea should not be consumed for a period longer than that which is instructed. In most occasions, the use of diet tea should not be for longer than two weeks.

Upon experiencing of side effects when using this tea, it is advisable to immediately discontinue use.

Do not take the tea in excess. Too much of this tea may produce unwanted negative health effects such as nausea, diarrhoea, abdominal discomfort and dehydration. For this reason, it is advised to limit your intake to just a cup.

Ensure that you follow the guidelines provided on the labels of the diet tea you purchase. This will ensure that one not only sees the positive benefits but avoids the negative effects of the diet tea.

Finally, keep the tea in a place away from children and that where it is cool and dry as well.

Frequently Asked Questions about Diets

If you have ever tried to lose weight and/or read through a million diet plans in the process, you probably have a few long standing questions.

Weight loss is important and is good (depending on your current weight of course) but being healthy is even more important.

You want to do it, but you definitely want to do it right. Eating cotton or paper to mimic fullness is not doing it right for one thing and can really affect your health.

Here are a few frequently asked questions about diets some people ask; some of which you might be asking yourself and their honest answers.

1. How Much Weight do I need to lose to make a difference?
If you have just hopped onto the weight loss wagon and your BMI is pretty much well over 30, you might be thinking you need to shed tons before your health problems go away.

The truth is losing only five percent of your current weight is enough to make an impact on your cholesterol, blood pressure and even your health risks with cancers and diabetes. Take heart; a little at a time is best.

2. Does starvation work?

Yes and no. Starving does not really do much for helping you lose weight in the long run. It will make you ravenous (literally) and irritable on top of thoroughly unhealthy.

You need to eat a balanced diet to give your body all the nutrients it needs. Far from giving you that bikini body you want, you will get a badly malnourished one.
As an added disadvantage, once you begin to feed yourself again, your fat will come piling right back on as your body initiates its failsafe for another starvation period.

Reducing your meal intake is far more effective.

3. Which diet plan is the best one for quick weight loss?

This is another very typical question. With so many diet plans out there, there are bound to be some that work for you but you really don't want to have to sift through the hundred and something others to find that one.

The best way of doing this is to get the expert advice of a doctor, nutritionist or fitness instructor/personal trainer. These people have adequate knowledge of how your body works and what is best for you.

Plus, if there is something you don't' like about your diet, you can ask them to switch things up for you and give you a whole new plan. Moreover, the plan suits you just right and is easy to pick up and stick to.

4. Do diet pills really work?

Yes and no. Diet pills have been on the receiving end of a lot of criticism and a lot of praise. The question of whether they really work or not more or less boils down to what you are using them for.

If you are using them on their own and expecting weight loss, you may be in for a rude shock. Diet pills are mainly supplementary to a diet and nothing more.

They may accelerate metabolism but only with exercise. They may promote fat loss if you use them as specified – with an exercise plan.

They may provide you with those nutrients you do not otherwise get or those you really need to curb side effects of a diet.

DO NOT use them to replace a healthy diet plan or exercise regimen. Consult a doctor before use.

5. Will taking more diet pills help me lose weight faster?

No. There is no "magic method" of losing weight fast. An overdose on diet pills is an overdose of medicine. Some already come with horrible side effects which will only be compounded (if they don't kill you first) with an overdose.

The reason there is a dosage is to help you lose weight appropriately. Moreover, it is not the pills that will let you lose weight, it is your dietary adjustments and exercise regimen.

The pills are only complementary to these and may or may not be included in a diet to make it effective.

6. If I am on a diet, do I need to exercise as well?

Diet and exercise go hand in hand for effective weight loss. One cannot really go without the other since they affect each other so much.

Think about it; if you still scarf down burgers, fries, pizzas and all those yummy but terribly unhealthy meals then run a mile, you may have kept the fat off but the cholesterol may get you in the end.

The reverse is also true. You need to work off the calories if you want to lose weight effectively and in the healthiest way.

7. With the right diet and exercise, how soon can I expect to see some results?

Depending on the diet in question, you may begin seeing results immediately although not necessarily in terms of weight loss.
Your energy levels may rise and your cravings may go down.

You may find yourself up and about without needing your coffee pick-me up in the morning. These little changes go a very long way in ensuring that you reach your weight loss goals effectively in the months to come and keep it off in the long run.

The really strict diets can see you lose up to 15lbs (7kg) in a week or two and progressively two to three pounds in the subsequent weeks.

8. What foods are bad for me?

There are certain foods that are considered unhealthy and not good for one on a diet. Some of these are genuinely not good for your health and others have added benefits you may like.

Chocolate for one thing is a great mood raiser and may have properties to help you with your weight loss, again depending on your diet.

Avocadoes have lots of fat but they contain essential fats which are much better for you than that bag of fries. They also have fiber which aids your digestive system. Doing your research is the key to figuring out which is which.

9. Why do I need to consult a doctor before trying my diet?

Your doctor pretty much understands where you are coming from and where you are heading. They also have your family history and personal medical history including allergic reactions on file.

Talking to a doctor before you begin a diet is possibly the best thing you can do.
Not only will they give you the best advice concerning your diet, but they also take into account your personal condition and have more insight on the contents of diet pills (if you want to start taking them).

Some of these pills, as mentioned also need a prescription so your doctor will also be able to let you know if you need them at all.

Books By Charlotte Wise

Series: Health & Fitness Ways To Improve Body & Mind

*Find Slim Body – Impressive Results Walking 5 Miles Daily at
http://www.amazon.com/dp/B00Q6QOE4U

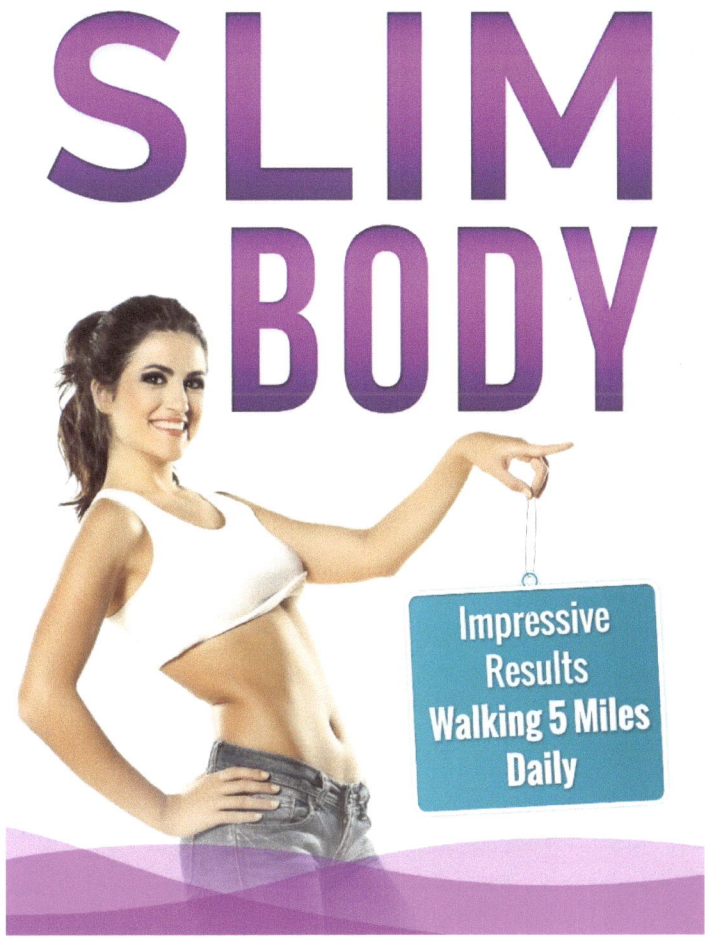

*Find The Healthy Smoothie Recipes Book – 70 Healthy & Nutritious Smoothie Recipes For Weight Loss, Diabetes, Blood Pressure And Much More at
http://www.amazon.com/dp/B00QL3PIO8

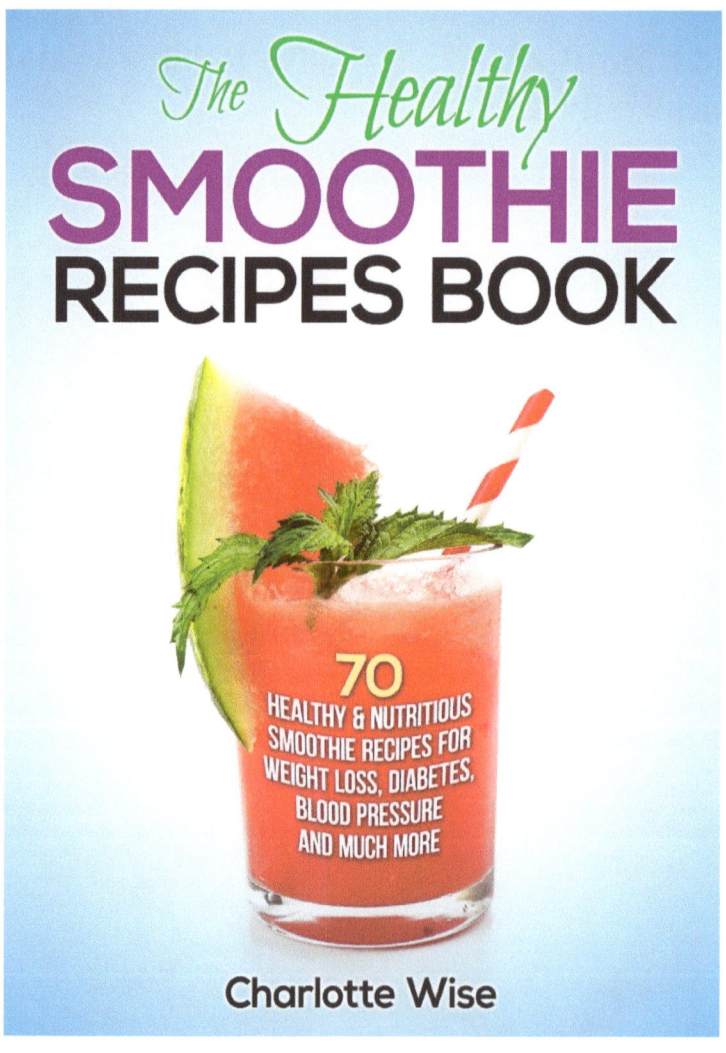

Quick favour please….

Take a minute to leave a review comment on Amazon letting me know if you have learned from this book.

I always want to hear from my readers and know how your healthy life is going.

Thanks and Good Luck ☺

Charlotte Wise